Beau
150 Simp
and Hair Care Recipes to Use Everyday

by **Vesela Tabakova**
Text copyright(c)2016 Vesela Tabakova

All rights reserved. No part of this publication may be reproduced, distributed, or transmitted in any form or by any means, including photocopying, recording, or other electronic or mechanical methods, without the prior written permission of the publisher, except in the case of brief quotations embodied in critical reviews and certain other noncommercial uses permitted by copyright law.

Although every precaution has been taken to verify the accuracy of the information contained herein, the author and publisher assume no responsibility for any errors or omissions. No liability is assumed for damages that may result from the use of information contained within.

It is important to note that all of these cosmetic recipes contain natural ingredients, but even natural ingredients can cause allergic reactions in some individuals.

It is imperative that you test any substance on a small area of skin before using it the recommended way. If any redness, swelling or sensitivity occurs within 20-30 minutes, discontinue use immediately and remove the substance well.

Please be advised that you are using these beauty recipes at your own risk. The author cannot be held liable or responsible for any reaction that you encounter while using any of these beauty recipes.

The idea, procedures and suggestions in this book are not intended as a substitute for consulting with your doctor and none of these formulations are meant to treat or diagnose any medical condition.

DxN1xBGcRRMA

Item Descriptions	Quantity
Beauty from Nature: 150 Simple Homemade Skin and Hair Care Recipes to Use Everyday: Organic Beauty on a Budget	1

https://www.amazon.ca/spr/returns/label/d9f41aac-909c-4a71-a88c-2639dbda0807?rmaId=DxN1xBGcRRMA&ref=ppx_yo2ov_dt_b_rtn_lbl

Table Of Contents

It is Easy to Be Beautiful!	8
Basic Ingredients of Homemade Skin and Hair Care Recipes	10
General Rules for Applying Homemade Face Scrubs and Masks	14
Face Scrubs and Body Exfoliants	15
Sweet Olive Oil Scrub	16
Flax Seed Scrub	16
Strawberry Exfoliant Scrub	16
Honey Scrub	17
Olive Oil and Salt Scrub	17
Baking Soda Scrub	17
Almond Scrub	18
Oatmeal Bran Scrub	18
Coffee Scrub	19
Tomato Scrub	19
Oatmeal-Aloe vera Scrub	19
Rice Flour Scrub	20
Orange and Honey Scrub	20
Banana Sensitive Skin Scrub	21
Body Exfoliants	22
Simple Coconut Body Scrub	22
Calming Chamomile and Vanilla Body Scrub	22
Thyme Body Scrub	23
Lemon Body Scrub	23
Oatmeal Body Scrub	23
Energizing Body Scrub	24
Relaxing Avocado Body Scrub	24
Oatmeal and Sea Salt Scrub	25
Peppermint Foot Scrub	25
Coconut Sugar Scrub	26
Cucumber Body Scrub	26
Peach Body Scrub	27
Mango Body Scrub	27
Coconut and Grapefruit Scrub	28
Tropical Scrub	28
Honey and Orange Scrub	29
Dry Skin Body Scrub	29
Lavender Body Scrub Recipe	30
Rosemary Body Scrub	30

Homemade Salt Scrub Recipe	31
Banana-Sugar Body Scrub	31
Coffee Body Scrub	32
Citrus Body Scrub	32
End of Summer Body Scrub	33
Autumn Body Scrub	33
Argan Oil Body Scrub	34
Face Masks	35
Strained Yogurt Mask	35
Yogurt and Parsley Mask	35
Whitening Yogurt Mask	36
Simple Yogurt Mask	36
Calming Yogurt Mask	36
Skin Brightener Yogurt Mask	37
Olive Oil Anti-wrinkle Mask	37
Oat Bran Face Mask	37
Rose Water Mask	39
Purifying Rose Water Mask	39
Pear Mask	40
Pear and Honey Mask	40
Toning Cucumber Mask	41
Honey and Cucumber Mask	41
Moisturizing Cucumber Mask	42
Dry Yeast Mask	42
Silky Skin Mask	42
Coffee and Cocoa Mask	43
Coffee Mask	43
Firming Coffee Mask	44
Raw Potato Mask	44
Potato and Cucumber Mask	45
Egg Yolk Mask	45
Cucumber and Strawberry Mask	46
Strawberry Face Mask	46
Acne Clearing Mask	47
Strawberry and Oats Mask	47
Banana Nourishing Mask	47
Calming Oat Mask	48
Almond Mask	48
Apple Anti-wrinkle Mask	49
Autumn Apple Mask	49

Reviving Avocado Mask	50
Avocado Mask	50
Nourishing Avocado Mask	51
Tomato and Avocado Mask	51
Honey and Milk Mask	52
Firming Face Mask	52
Honey and Clay Mask	52
White Clay Mask	53
Lifting Honey and Clay Mask	53
Anti-aging Red Wine Face Mask	54
Wheat Bran Mask	54
Peach Mask	54
Peach and Honey Mask	55
Homemade Face Creams and Lotions	56
Best Kept Secrets for Healthy Hair	58
Hair Growing Tips	60
Nutrition for a Healthy Hair Growth	64
Centuries-old Tips on How to Use the Moon to Grow Your Hair	66
General Rules for Applying Homemade Hair Masks	66
Basic Ingredients of Homemade Hair Shampoos, Masks and Conditioners	68
Natural Homemade Shampoos	71
Baking Soda Wash	72
Egg Yolk Shampoo	72
Tea Tree Oil Shampoo	72
Pomegranate Oil Shampoo	72
Lemon and Egg Shampoo	72
Avocado Shampoo	73
Moisturizing Egg Shampoo	73
Yogurt Shampoo	73
Homemade Hair Treatments that Stimulate Hair Growth	74
Oatmeal Hair Mask	75
Burdock Hair Mask	75
Burdock Root Rinse	75
Vitamin A Hair Mask	76
Mustard Hair Mask	76
Castor Oil Mask	77
Rosemary Rinse	77
Almond Oil Treatment	77
Nettle Hair Rinse	78

Lemon Juice and Coriander Leaves	78
Onions for Long Hair	79
Egg and Onion Mask	79
Green Tea and Tea Tree Oil	79
Potato and Aloe Vera Hair Mask	80
Cinnamon Honey Mask	80
Beer and Egg Hair Mask	80
Egg Yolk and Honey	80
Treatments to Get Rid of Dandruff	82
Thyme Dandruff Treatment	83
Thyme Hair Rinse	83
Strawberry Dandruff Mask	83
Camphor Oil Mask for Dandruff	83
Camphor Rinse	84
Coconut Lemon Mask	84
Ginger Dandruff Treatment	84
The Best Homemade Hair Masks	85
Masks for Dry Hair	86
Warm Oil Treatment	86
Nourishing Cocoa Mask	86
Coconut Mask	87
Simple Dry Hair Banana Mask	87
Sweet Banana Mask	87
Banana Avocado Hair Mask	88
Avocado Dry Hair Mask	88
Dry Hair Egg Mask	88
Masks for Oily Hair	89
Basic Mask for Oily Hair	89
Baking Soda Mask	89
Yogurt Mask for Oily Hair	89
Honey and Apple Cider Mask for Oily Hair	91
Strawberry Hair Mask for Oily Hair	91
Avocado Mask for Oily Hair	91
Simple Clay Mask	91
Egg Yolk and Clay Mask for Oily Hair	92
Nettle Rinse	93
Walnut Leaves Rinse	93
Lavender Water Rinse	94
Apple Cider Vinegar Rinse	94
Coffee or Black Tea Hair Rinse	94

Masks for Combination Hair	95
Masks for Normal Hair	95
Milk and Honey Mask	95
A Nourishing Normal Hair Mask	95
Beer Treatment for Normal Hair	96
Beer Rinse	96
Regenerating Mask	96
Coconut Oil Mask	96
Clay Mask for Normal Hair	97
About the Author	98

It is Easy to Be Beautiful!

Today more and more people are starting to realize we are surrounded with harmful chemicals and although our lives have become easier, we are paying a high price for this convenience. As we are getting more and more informed we find out that many common cosmetic products are actually bad for our health and can even cause terrible sicknesses. Most commercially produced cosmetics contain preservatives and ingredients that cause more harm than good for the body. We are slowly discovering that making small changes in our lifestyles can significantly improve our quality of life and health.

The most important benefit from making our own cosmetic products is that we can control what goes in and, therefore, we can use only clean, organic, natural, chemical-free ingredients and stay away from the harmful ones.

Although preparing homemade facial scrubs and masks may seem as if we are rejecting progress, it is actually the best way to maintain beautifully young and healthy skin with very little effort.

The recipes I have included in this book are well known in Bulgaria and have been used from almost every woman at some point in time. Most are very easy to follow and can be prepared in a few minutes with products everyone has in the kitchen. The best part is it usually doesn't cost a thing because we already have fruit, vegetables, olive oil, dairy, oats, coffee and cocoa at home. Many of the masks and scrubs involve simply mixing together a few ingredients and gently massaging them on the face, neck and, why not, the hands.

These recipes do not contain any artificial fragrances or colors, nor do they need preservatives, because they are intended for immediate use. They are suitable for all skin types. However, please be aware that if you have a known food allergy, chances are you will be allergic to a cosmetic product made from the same food. Care should always be taken when using a new product - be sure to test a small area for skin sensitivity before using any mixture on your face. Dab a little on the inside of your wrist or the underside of your arm and wait a 24 to see if it causes a reaction, such as a rash.

Face Scrubs

As we age, skin cells die and form a build-up due to the slowing down of collagen and elastin production. This build-up can have the effect of blocking skin pores and causing signs of aging. Scrubs act on the skin like fine-grained sandpaper on wood. They exfoliate dead skin cells and leave only the newer and healthy skin cells. In this way face skin appears vital and fresh. After cleaning the skin with a gentle scrub it is more ready for the absorption of other skin treatments like nourishing face masks and moisturizers. There is debate about the frequency of use of scrubs as exfoliators, but it is generally thought that this should be adjusted based on skin response. Some skin types may need scrubs only once a week, whereas oilier skin may need scrubs as frequently as on alternate days. In oily-to-normal skin types, exfoliation with scrubs can be carried out 3–4 times a week. Individuals with dry skin should restrict the use of exfoliating scrubs to once or twice a week.

Masks

Homemade masks work by doing several things to our skin – they draw blood to its surface, provide essential nutrients to dull, lifeless, and aging skin. A nice homemade face mask will not only enhance the look of your skin, it will make you feel good and beautiful. Cleaning and moisturizing your skin regularly will make its texture brighter and more translucent.

By using gifts from nature like yogurt, eggs, honey, oats, common fruit and vegetables, Bulgarian Rose essential oil and Rose water, different types of clay and herbs every woman, no matter what age, can achieve healthy, young looking skin and good overall health.

Basic Ingredients of Homemade Skin and Hair Care Recipes

Yogurt is one of the best homemade beauty ingredients because it's full of protein, calcium, vitamins D and B and probiotics. Lactic acid, a natural alpha hydroxy acid, in yogurt helps smooth and exfoliate skin. When topically applied to the skin as a facial mask, yogurt moisturizes, fights acne, prevents premature aging, relieves sunburn and reduces discoloration. In Bulgaria where I live women commonly use yogurt as a facial mask and it probably is one of the secrets of the famous Bulgarian beauty.

The **Bulgarian Rose Essential Oil** is one of the safest oils suitable for all skin types. It is produced from the precious and beautiful *Rosa damascena* flowers grown in The Valley of the Roses in Bulgaria and is one of the most expensive essential oils because it takes about 3000-3500 kg of rose petals to distill only one kilogram of rose oil. Bulgarian rose oil is famous for its antibacterial, antidepressant, anti fungal, antimicrobial, antiseptic, astringent and deodorant properties.

Bulgarian Rose Water helps stimulate the flow in the minute blood vessels under the skin and helps heal scars, minor infections, sunburn, and damaged skin. It is a natural mild antiseptic and can help relieve acne and other skin conditions. Rose water can also be applied to insect bites and sunburns.

Honey is a natural antioxidant and is well known for its anti-microbial properties. It supports the skin's ability to rejuvenate and refresh and also absorbs impurities from the pores on the skin, making it an ideal cleansing agent.

Ground oats and ***oats bran*** are soothing and gentle on the skin. They are good skin cleansers and are especially great for dry and irritated skin. Oatmeal has long been used to help alleviate irritated skin, skin rashes, and other conditions that cause itching. It is excellent in scrubs and masks for all skin types, including acne-prone and sensitive skin.

Cucumbers are rich in fiber and contain a variety of beneficial minerals, including silica, potassium and magnesium. The silica which is found in cucumber's skin is an essential component of healthy connective tissue, which includes muscles, tendons, ligaments, cartilage, and bones. Cucumber's high water content makes it naturally hydrating and cucumber juice is often recommended as a source of silica to improve the complexion and health of the skin. The natural ascorbic acid and caffeic acid within the cucumber act to prevent water retention in the skin. This reduces swelling under the eyes and helps the skin heal from sunburn, inflammation, and eczema. Cucumbers are typically highly sprayed with pesticides, so it is always better to get organic varieties.

Raw potatoes are rich in minerals such as Potassium, Sulfur and Phosphorous which are excellent for skin care as well as vitamins and antioxidant compounds. It has long been known that raw potato juice, helps improve the skin tone. Potatoes also help control and prevent acne, pimples and blackheads, soothe the inflammation on skin wounds, reduce the appearance of eye bags under the eyes and clears skin by cleansing the excess oil from the skin.

Strawberries are high in vitamin C and also contain a high amount of other vitamins and minerals. The antioxidants in strawberries help the skin fight off damaging free radicals from the sun, stress and pollution. Salicylic acid found in strawberries can help get rid of dead skin cells. Strawberries are also known for whitening skin and protecting it from diseases. Like potatoes and cucumbers, they can be a key ingredient in helping reduce dark circles under the eyes.

Bananas are one of the most nourishing fruits available because they contain large quantities of magnesium, potassium, zinc, iodine, iron and vitamins A, B, E, and F, and much more. Because of these qualities bananas are often used to battle dry skin and wrinkles. Banana-based facials masks moisturize and soothe the skin.

Avocados are compatible with most skin types. They are full of beta carotene, vitamins B, C and E, and are also packed with protein and natural oils.

Egg products can help smooth lines and prevent fine wrinkles. Egg whites are great for firming the skin and are used in a lot of anti-aging face masks.

Olive oil nourishes and smooths the skin. It is full of poly phenol antioxidants which help to undo the damage of sun, free radicals and pollution. Olive oil also is one of my favorite natural face moisturizers.

Aloe vera gel comes from the Aloe vera plant. It is perfect for all skin types and is effective in soothing the skin and reducing inflammation, sunburns and rashes. Aloe vera gel can even help skin with acne because it has antibacterial and anti-inflammatory properties that reduce skin inflammation. It allows the skin to heal naturally with minimal scarring. Aloe vera is a good moisturizing ingredient in a lot of face masks because it doesn't give the skin a greasy feel.

Milk is good for soothing mild sunburn and some shaving irritations.

White clay draws impurities from the skin and unclogs pores.

Almonds are a gentle exfoliant and promote healthy skin.

Baking soda soothes itchy skin and helps clear complexion.

Sugar, brown or white, is a good exfoliant and circulation stimulator.

Sea salt promotes circulation and exfoliation. You can use table salt too.

Lemon or lime juice is a natural astringent and restores pH balance for oily skin. It opens pores. *Lemons* are great for lightening dark spots on the skin.

Apple cider vinegar is fermented apple juice. It is packed with natural minerals like magnesium, calcium, iron and phosphorus. It helps restore skin's acid balance.

General Rules for Applying Homemade Face Scrubs and Masks

The usual rules of skin care apply while using masks and scrubs to derive optimal results:

Pull back hair, tie it and get it out of the way.

Remove make-up regularly and completely every day.

Wash skin well before applying a facial mask. Exfoliate with home prepared scrubs rather than commercial ones.

Scrubs should not be used by individuals experiencing an active outbreak of acne because they can aggravate the problem and introduce infection. Also don't scrub if you have an active infection, cold sore, sunburn, extremely dry skin, redness or inflammation for any reason. Let skin heal first.

Scrubbing should be done gently with fingertips in a circular motion, ideally in the shower or right before going into the shower.

Fresh face scrubs are the best, it is better to make a face scrub just enough for one time use.

Body scrubs contain oil and can make the tub or shower slippery. Be extra careful as you may slip. Be sure to wash well the tub when you're done.

Always apply masks with fingertips or a gentle brush. Apply masks over the forehead, cheeks, nose, chin and neck - never around the eye area because it is really sensitive.

Try to relax when you have put a mask on.

Fresh masks are the best, it is better to make a face mask just enough for one time use.

Face Scrubs and Body Exfoliants

Sweet Olive Oil Scrub

Ingredients:

1 tbsp olive oil

1/2 tbsp honey

1 tbsp brown sugar

Directions:

Mix olive oil and honey in a small cup. Add sugar to the mixture and stir well. Wet face, and rub onto face and neck then rinse with warm water.

Flax Seed Scrub

Ingredients:

1 tsp dry milk

1 tsp honey

1 tsp flax seeds

Directions:

Combine all ingredients in a small cup. Wet face, and gently wash it with the scrub.

Strawberry Exfoliant Scrub

Ingredients:

1 tsp sea salt

3 strawberries

1 tsp olive oil

Directions:

Mix together strawberries, salt and olive oil. Scrub face and neck, rinse, pat dry and moisturize.

Honey Scrub

Ingredients:

1 tbsp honey

1 tsp lemon juice

1 tsp sugar

Directions:

Mix 1 tbsp of honey with 1 teaspoon of lemon juice and one teaspoon of sugar in a small bowl.

Rinse your face with fresh water and scrub face for one minute. Wash with cool water.

Olive Oil and Salt Scrub

Ingredients:

1 tbsp olive oil

1 tsp very finely ground sea salt

Directions:

Mix the two ingredients in a small bowl. Scrub your face for two minutes and then wash with warm water.

Baking Soda Scrub

Ingredients:

1 tsp baking soda

1 tsp honey

1 tsp olive oil

Directions:

Mix the ingredients into a paste.

Using your fingertips in a circular motion, apply to face and gently scrub for a minute then rinse.

Almond Scrub

Ingredients:

1 tbsp plain yogurt

1 tsp finely ground almonds.

2 drops Bulgarian rose essential oil

Directions:

Mix well into a paste and scrub face for two minutes.

Wash with warm water.

Oatmeal Bran Scrub

Ingredients:

1 tbsp oatmeal bran

1 tbsp yogurt

1 tsp lemon juice

Directions:

Combine ingredients in a bowl and apply with fingertips.

Leave for one minute, scrub, and rinse with lukewarm water.

Coffee Scrub

Ingredients:

1 tsp very fine coffee grounds

½ tsp olive oil

Directions:

Mix the two ingredients and apply gently to face and massage with fingertips in circular motion.

Rinse with warm water.

Tomato Scrub

Ingredients:

1 small tomato

1 tsp fine granulated sugar

Directions:

Mash tomato pulp with a fork and mix it with sugar.

Massage on to face, wait two minutes and rinse.

Oatmeal-Aloe vera Scrub

Ingredients:

2 tbsp finely ground oatmeal

1 tsp honey

1/2 tsp olive oil

1/2 tsp Aloe vera gel

1 tsp water

Directions:

Mix all ingredients in a small bowl. Apply to face and neck with gentle, circular strokes, leave for about a minute.

Rinse with cool water and pat dry.

Rice Flour Scrub

Ingredients:

2 tbsp of rice powder

1 tbsp rose water

1 tbsp lemon juice

Directions:

Mix and stir ingredients well to form a paste. Gently apply to face and scrub for a minute.

Wash off with lukewarm water.

Orange and Honey Scrub

Ingredients:

Ingredients:

1 tbsp finely ground oatmeal

1 tsp orange zest

1 tbsp honey

1 tbsp water

Directions:

Combine all ingredients in a small bowl and mix together well. Gently apply the scrub on your face and massage for 1-2 minutes.

Rinse, pat dry and moisturize.

Banana Sensitive Skin Scrub

Ingredients:

½ banana, mashed

1 tbsp oatmeal

Directions:

Mash half banana with a fork and mix it with the oatmeal.

Gently massage onto skin for a minute then rinse off.

Body Exfoliants

Simple Coconut Body Scrub

Ingredients:

1 cup brown sugar

1/2 cup coconut oil

1/2 tsp vanilla extract

Directions:

Mix half a cup of coconut oil with one cup of brown sugar. Add a tsp of vanilla extract.

Apply the mixture to damp skin. Gently exfoliate in small, circular motions. Rinse with warm water.

Calming Chamomile and Vanilla Body Scrub

Ingredients:

1/2 cup brown sugar

2 tbsp dried chamomile buds

1 tsp vanilla extract

1 tbsp honey

3 tbsp olive oil

Directions:

Combine vanilla and sugar until well mixed. Add the chamomile buds, crushing them slightly between your fingers. Stir in the olive oil, the honey, and mix until evenly combined.

Gently massage on body and scrub with circular motions. Rinse with warm water and pat dry.

Thyme Body Scrub

Ingredients:

1/2 cup sugar

5 tbsp olive oil

2 tbsp dried thyme leaves

Directions:

Combine sugar and thyme leaves. Add olive oil and stir well. Apply the mixture to damp skin.

Gently exfoliate in small, circular motions. Rinse with warm water.

Lemon Body Scrub

Ingredients:

1/2 cup sugar

4 tbsp almond oil

1 tbsp lemon juice

1 tbsp lemon zest

1-2 drops Lemon Essential Oil

Directions:

Mix all ingredients and apply the mixture to damp skin. Gently exfoliate in small, circular motions.

Rinse with warm water and pat dry.

Oatmeal Body Scrub

Ingredients:

½ cup oatmeal, coarsely ground

2 tbsp honey

1 tbsp apple cider vinegar

2 tbsp olive oil

1 drop Bulgarian rose Oil

Directions:

Stir ingredients until you make a smooth paste. Add 1 drop of Bulgarian Rose oil to the mixture. Apply the mixture to damp skin.

Gently exfoliate in small, circular motions. Rinse with warm water and pat dry.

Energizing Body Scrub

Ingredients:

1/2 cup brown sugar

5 tbsp grapeseed oil

3 tbsp orange zest

Directions:

Mix sugar and orange zest. Add the grapeseed oil and stir until well combined.

Apply the mixture to damp skin. Gently exfoliate in small, circular motions. Rinse with warm water.

Relaxing Avocado Body Scrub

Ingredients:

1 cup oatmeal, coarsely ground

½ cup avocado oil

4-5 drops lavender essential oil

Directions:

Mix all ingredients in a glass bowl or jar.

Rub into damp skin, massage for 2-3 minutes and rinse with warm water.

Oatmeal and Sea Salt Scrub

Ingredients:

1/3 cup ground oatmeal

1/3 cup sea salt

½ cup grapeseed oil

4-5 drops Bulgarian Rose Essential Oil

Directions:

Mix salt, oatmeal and oil in a clean, glass bowl. Stir well with a spoon. Add a few drops of Bulgarian Rose Essential Oil.

Rub into damp skin, massage for 2-3 minutes and rinse off.

Peppermint Foot Scrub

Ingredients:

1/3 cup sea salt

1/3 cup baking soda

4-5 tbsp olive oil

15 drops peppermint oil

5 drops tea tree oil

Directions:

Mix salt and baking soda, gradually add olive oil and stir until you have a slightly wet, but grainy consistency. Add the Peppermint Essential Oil and Tea Tree Oil.

Massage the homemade foot scrub in a circular motion into bottoms of feet. Rinse and dry feet.

Coconut Sugar Scrub

Ingredients:

1 cup brown sugar

1/4 cup coconut oil

3 tbsp shredded coconut

4-5 drops Lemon Essential Oil

Directions:

Mix brown sugar with shredded coconut. Add coconut oil and mix. Add a few drops of Lemon Essential Oil.

Apply to damp skin and gently exfoliate. Rinse with warm water.

Cucumber Body Scrub

Ingredients:

1/2 cucumber, unpeeled, pureed (½ cup)

1 cup raw sugar

4 tbsp almond oil

Directions:

Cut and blend half cucumber until smooth. Add it to the sugar and add 4 tablespoons of almond oil. Mix until well blended.

Gently exfoliate in small, circular motions. Rinse with warm water.

Peach Body Scrub

Ingredients:

1 ripe peach, unpeeled, mashed

1/2 cup sugar

4 tbsp olive oil

Directions:

Combine ingredients in a glass bowl and mix together until smooth.

Apply scrub to damp skin and massage gently all over your body. Rinse with warm water.

Mango Body Scrub

Ingredients:

1/2 cup sugar

½ cup ground oats

1/2 cup mango puree

1/2 cup coconut oil

2 tbsp lemon juice

Directions:

Peel and blend mango to puree. Mix sugar, oatmeal and coconut oil in a glass bowl.

Stir well to combine then add in lemon juice and mango puree.

Apply to wet body and massage in circular motion. Rinse with warm water.

Coconut and Grapefruit Scrub

Ingredients:

½ cup sugar

2 tbsp shredded coconut

2 tbsp jojoba oil

1 tbsp olive oil

2 tbsp fresh grapefruit juice

2 drops grapefruit essential oil

Directions:

In a glass bowl or jar, combine sugar, shredded coconut, grapefruit juice, olive oil and jojoba oil. Add grapefruit essential oil and stir well to combine.

Gently exfoliate in small, circular motions. Rinse with warm water.

Tropical Scrub

Ingredients:

1 cup sugar

2 tbsp sesame seeds

5 tbsp coconut oil

2 tbsp fresh orange juice

2 drops Orange Essential Oil

Directions:

Mix sugar, sesame seeds and coconut oil in a glass bowl. Stir to combine and add remaining ingredients.

Gently exfoliate in circular motions. Rinse with warm water.

Honey and Orange Scrub

Ingredients:

1 cup coarsely ground oatmeal

5 tbsp honey

3 tbsp fresh orange juice

Directions:

In a glass bowl or jar, mix all ingredients until smooth.

Massage and gently exfoliate in small, circular motions. Rinse with warm water.

Dry Skin Body Scrub

Ingredients:

½ cup brown sugar

½ cup sea salt salt

2-3 tbsp honey

2 tbsp argan oil

2 tbsp fresh orange juice

Directions:

Mix all ingredients until you have a smooth paste. Apply to wet skin and exfoliate body in small, circular motions.

Rinse with warm water.

Lavender Body Scrub Recipe

Ingredients:

1/2 cup sugar

2 tbsp lavender leaves

¼ cup jojoba oil

3 drops lavender essential oil

Directions:

Combine sugar and lavender leaves. Add jojoba oil and lavender essential oil. Apply the mixture to damp skin.

Gently exfoliate in small, circular motions. Rinse with warm water.

Rosemary Body Scrub

Ingredients:

1/2 cup coconut oil

1/2 cup sugar

1/4 cup flax seeds

7-8 drops Rosemary Essential Oil

Directions:

Combine sugar and flax seeds and stir until mixed well. Add the coconut oil and mix until evenly combined. Apply the mixture to damp skin.

Gently exfoliate in small, circular motions. Rinse with warm water.

Homemade Salt Scrub Recipe

Ingredients:

1/2 cup salt

3 tbsp ground coffee

2 tbsp honey

¼ cup avocado oil

1 tsp of vanilla extract

Directions:

Combine salt and ground coffee. Add honey and avocado oil and stir until smooth. Add vanilla extract and apply to damp skin.

Gently exfoliate in small, circular motions. Rinse with warm water.

Banana-Sugar Body Scrub

Ingredients:

1 ripe banana

4 tbsp raw sugar

1 tbsp cocoa powder

2 tbsp almond oil

¼ tsp pure vanilla extract

Directions:

Smash ingredients together with a fork.

Gently massage over your body for a few minutes. Rinse off with warm water

Coffee Body Scrub

Ingredients:

1/4 cup ground coffee

1/4 cup sugar

3 tbsp olive oil

1 vitamin E capsule

Directions:

Mix sugar with ground coffee, olive oil and the Vitamin E capsule.

Apply over wet body and massage gently. Rinse off with warm water.

Citrus Body Scrub

Ingredients:

1/2 cup of brown sugar

1 tbsp of lemon juice

1 tbsp lemon zest

2 tbsp olive oil

Directions:

Mix all the ingredients well. Moisten your skin, massage and scrub gently all over your body.

Rinse with warm water and pat dry.

End of Summer Body Scrub

Ingredients:

1/3 cup ground flax seeds

1/3 cup oatmeal, coarsely ground

1/2 cup yogurt

1 tbsp olive oil

Directions:

Combine flax seeds and oatmeal. Add yogurt and olive oil and stir. Gently exfoliate in small, circular motions.

Rinse with warm water.

Autumn Body Scrub

Ingredients:

1/3 cup pureed pumpkin

1/2 cup brown sugar

2 tbsp honey

1 tbsp olive oil

½ tsp cinnamon

½ tsp nutmeg

Directions:

Mix pureed pumpkin with sugar, honey and olive oil and stir to combine. Add cinnamon and nutmeg and stir some more.

Apply scrub on damp skin and massage gently for 5 minutes. Rinse with warm water and pat dry.

Argan Oil Body Scrub

Ingredients:

1/2 cup brown sugar

2 tbsp honey

2 tbsp argan oil

3-5 drops of Rosemary Essential Oil

Directions:

Mix the Argan Oil into the sugar and honey and stir until smooth. Add 4 drops of Rosemary Essential Oil.

Massage onto damp skin and scrub for several minutes. Wash with warm water.

Face Masks

Strained Yogurt Mask

Ingredients:

5 tbsp plain yogurt

1 slice of white bread

Directions:

This is a very old family recipe and is also the easiest basic face mask. It was used probably by every Bulgarian mother and grandmother back in the days when there were no commercial creams and moisturizers.

Place the slice of bread in a plate, put the yogurt on top of it, spread it evenly and leave in the fridge for a few hours or overnight.

In the morning take the strained yogurt and spread it on your clean face – leave it for 20 minutes and rinse it with water. Results are always excellent.

Yogurt and Parsley Mask

Ingredients:

5 tbsp pain yogurt

2 tbsp fresh parsley finely cut

Directions:

Strain the yogurt over a slice of bread for a few hours (see above), then mix it with the finely cut parsley and apply on your face in a thick layer.

Leave for 20 minutes and rinse with lukewarm water.

Whitening Yogurt Mask

Ingredients:

2 tbsp plain yogurt

1 tbsp finely ground oats

Directions:

Mix yogurt and oats well and spread on face and neck. After it goes dry wash with warm water.

Simple Yogurt Mask

Ingredients:

1 tbsp plain yogurt

1 tbsp honey

Directions:

Stir well the two ingredients and apply to your face. Wash after 15 minutes.

Calming Yogurt Mask

Ingredients:

2 tbsp plain yogurt

1 large Aloe vera leaf

Directions:

Take a large Aloe vera leaf from an aloe plant and squeeze out 1 tbsp of the gel into a small bowl.

Mix well yogurt and Aloe vera juice and apply to face. Leave for 10-15 minutes then rinse with lukewarm water.

Skin Brightener Yogurt Mask

Ingredients:

1tbsp of plain yogurt

1 tsp lemon juice

Directions:

Mix lemon juice with yogurt well.

Apply mask, and leave on for 5-10 minutes, then rinse off with warm water.

Olive Oil Anti-wrinkle Mask

Ingredients:

1 tbsp olive oil

1 tbsp lemon juice

Directions:

Mix well equal parts of lemon juice and olive oil and leave on face for ten minutes. For best results use twice a week.

Oat Bran Face Mask

Ingredients:

3 tbsp oats bran

hot water

2 drops Bulgarian rose essential oil

Directions:

Boil bran in ½ cup of water. Strain, cool add rose oil and apply to face. Leave for 15 minutes and wash with lukewarm water.

Rose Water Mask

Ingredients:

2 tbsp oatmeal

1 tbsp Rose water

1 tbsp honey

1 tsp plain yogurt

2 drops Bulgarian rose oil essential oil

Directions:

Combine the oatmeal, Rose water, honey and yogurt. Stir well and wait until the the mixture becomes creamy.

Add the rose oil last then spread the mask over your face and neck and leave it for 10 minutes.

When the mask starts to dry, rinse with warm water.

Purifying Rose Water Mask

Ingredients:

2 tbsp white clay

2 tbsp Rose water

1 drop Bulgarian rose essential oil

Directions:

Combine Rose water and clay in a glass bowl. Stir well and add the rose oil.

Apply to face and leave it until it starts to dry then gently wash off.

Pear Mask

Ingredients:

1 ripe pear

1 tsp sour cream

1 tbsp grapefruit juice

Directions:

Peel and cut the pear in a small bowl. Mash it very well with a fork then add the cream and the grapefruit juice.

Apply on your face and keep it on for 15 minutes, then rinse with water.

Pear and Honey Mask

Ingredients:

1 ripe pear

1 tbsp honey

1 tsp sour cream

Directions:

Peel and cut the pear, then mash it with a fork into a smooth paste. Stir in a tablespoon of honey and a teaspoon of cream.

Spread the mixture evenly over your face and neck. Leave it for 10 minutes then rinse off.

Toning Cucumber Mask

Ingredients:

3-4 leafs of fresh mint

1/2 cucumber

1 egg white.

Directions:

Peel the cucumber. Blend it along with the mint leaves into a puree. Beat the egg white and then add to the cucumber mixture.

Apply the mask evenly on your face for 20 minutes and then rinse it with water.

Honey and Cucumber Mask

Ingredients:

½ cucumber

1 egg white

1 tsp olive oil

1 tsp honey

2 tbsp finely powdered oats

Directions:

Combine all ingredients in a bowl and blend until you make a smooth paste.

Use your fingers to apply a thick layer of the mask to clean face and neck area and leave for 15 minutes. Rinse off with warm water.

Moisturizing Cucumber Mask

Ingredients:

1 tsp nonfat dry milk

¼ peeled cucumber

1 tbsp plain yogurt

2 drops of Bulgarian rose essential oil

Directions:

Put first three ingredients into a blender and mix well until creamy. Add two drops of rose oil and stir well.

Apply to your face avoiding eye area. Leave on for 15 minutes, then rinse off.

Dry Yeast Mask

Ingredients:

15 g active dry yeast

Directions:

Dilute yeast in warm or milk water until it becomes creamy.

Massage on face and leave until it dries then wash with lukewarm water.

Silky Skin Mask

Ingredients:

1 tsp fresh yeast

1 tsp milk

Directions:

Mix well slightly warm milk with 1 tsp fresh yeast until it gets creamy.

Apply to face with fingers and leave for 10 minutes then wash with lukewarm water.

Coffee and Cocoa Mask

Ingredients:

1 tsp very finely ground coffee beans

1 tsp cocoa powder

1 tbsp milk

Directions:

Mix together the ground coffee and cocoa powder in small cup. Add the milk and stir to achieve a creamy texture.

Spread on clean face and neck, avoiding eye and mouth area. Leave for 5 minutes. Rinse well with warm water.

Coffee Mask

Ingredients:

1 tbsp very finely ground coffee

1 tbsp olive oil

½ tbsp honey

Directions:

Mix together the ingredients, spread on clean face and neck, leave for 10 minutes, and then rinse well with warm water.

Firming Coffee Mask

Ingredients:

1 tsp used coffee grounds

1 tsp honey

1 tsp sour cream

2 egg whites

Directions:

Whip the egg whites then add sour cream, honey and coffee.

Spread on your clean face and neck, avoiding eye and mouth area and leave for 10 minutes. Wash with warm water.

Raw Potato Mask

Ingredients:

1 medium potato

1 tsp plain flour

1 tsp plain yogurt

Directions:

Grate potato, skin and all, strain it with the help of a cheese cloth. Mix the pulp with the flour and yogurt, stir well and apply to face.

Leave it for 15 minutes and clean with a moistened tissue then rinse with water.

Potato and Cucumber Mask

Ingredients:

1 medium raw potato

½ cucumber

1 egg yolk

1 tbsp plain yogurt

Directions:

Peel and blend potato and cucumber, add 1 egg yolk and 1 tbsp yogurt, make it into a fine paste and apply it to clean face.

Keep it on for 20 minutes before removing it and washing with warm water.

Egg Yolk Mask

Ingredients:

1 egg yolk

½ tsp honey

10 drops lemon juice

½ tsp finely ground oats

1 drops Bulgarian rose essential oil

Directions:

Beat egg yolk with honey, add lemon juice and rose oil, then thicken with half a teaspoon of finely ground oats.

Spread a thin layer on face and wash with lukewarm water after 15 minutes.

Cucumber and Strawberry Mask

Ingredients:

½ cucumber

2-3 strawberries

1 tsp plain yogurt

1 tsp oats bran

Directions:

Mix everything and blend with a blender to reach a cream-like texture.

Spread on clean face and leave until it dries. Wash with cool water.

Strawberry Face Mask

Ingredients:

3 strawberries

½ banana

1 tsp honey

Directions:

Mix strawberries, banana, and a tsp of honey in a blender. Blend it until all ingredients are in a smooth liquid.

Apply to your entire face and neck. Leave it on for about 15-20 minutes then wash with warm water.

Acne Clearing Mask

Ingredients:

½ cup strawberries

1 tbsp yogurt

Directions:

Mash together ½ cup fresh strawberries with 1 tbsp yogurt, spread on clean face, let sit for 15 minutes, and then rinse well.

Strawberry and Oats Mask

Ingredients:

2 large strawberries

1 tsp finely ground oats

1 tsp honey

Directions:

Blend strawberries with oats and honey in a food processor until you get a paste like mixture.

Spread it in a thick layer onto face and neck area with fingertips. Rest for 15-20 minutes. Rinse off with cool water.

Banana Nourishing Mask

Ingredients:

1 banana

1 tsp honey

1 tsp plain yogurt

Directions:

Mash a banana; add the honey and the yogurt; mix well and spread it evenly on a clean face.

Leave it for at least 15 minutes and wash with cold water.

Calming Oat Mask

Ingredients:

1 tbsp finely ground oats

1 tsp olive oil

1 tsp whole milk

Directions:

Mix a tablespoon of finely ground oats with a teaspoon of olive oil and a teaspoon of whole milk until the mixture is a paste.

Massage the paste into the skin and leave it for a few minutes before rinsing with cool to lukewarm water.

Almond Mask

Ingredients:

3 tsp almond flour or finely ground almonds

1 tsp honey

1 tsp sour cream

Directions:

Mix all three ingredients with a little warm water and apply to face. Wash after 15 minutes.

Apple Anti-wrinkle Mask

Ingredients:

1 apple

1 tsp lemon juice

1-2 drops Bulgarian rose essential oil

Directions:

Peel an apple and place into a blender. Add one teaspoon of lemon juice. Pulse until finely pureed.

Add the Rose oil and apply a thin layer to face. Rinse with cool water. For best results use once a week.

Autumn Apple Mask

Ingredients:

½ apple

1 tsp oatmeal

1 tsp honey

Directions:

Take a ripe ½ apple, grate it and mash it with a fork. Add one teaspoon oatmeal and 1 teaspoon honey to it and stir well.

Spread on face and leave it on until the mixture dries completely then rinse it off with ordinary water.

Reviving Avocado Mask

Ingredients:

½ avocado

2 tsp honey

1 tsp lemon juice

Directions:

Mash the avocado until it is smooth. Add the lemon, honey and stir well to create a smooth paste.

Spread over clean face and neck and leave it on for 15 minutes. Rinse well with warm water.

Avocado Mask

Ingredients:

1 ripe avocado

5-6 drops of lemon juice

2-3 drops of Bulgarian rose essential oil

Directions:

Mash one ripe avocado with 5-6 drops of lemon juice. Pour in a bowl and add 2-3 drops of Bulgarian rose essential oil, mix well and spread evenly onto clean face and neck.

Allow to stay on skin for 15 minutes then remove with cool water.

Nourishing Avocado Mask

Ingredients:

½ avocado

1 tbsp honey

1 tbsp apple vinegar

1 tbsp olive oil

Directions:

Mix avocado, honey and apple vinegar well. Stir, and add the olive oil.

Massage into face and leave for 30 minutes then rinse with lukewarm water.

Tomato and Avocado Mask

Ingredients:

½ tomato

1 avocado

1 tbsp lemon juice

1 tsp cornstarch

Directions:

Mash avocado with a fork in a small bowl. Cut and mash tomato with a fork then mix it with the avocado, add 1 tbsp lemon juice and 1 tsp cornstarch.

Combine everything well and apply a thick layer on face. Leave the mask for 30 minutes and rinse off.

Honey and Milk Mask

Ingredients:

1 tsp honey

3 tsp milk

½ cucumber

5 drops of fresh squeezed lemon juice

Directions:

Mix all the ingredients together thoroughly and gently massage the mask onto your face with fingers.

Leave on for 15 minutes then rinse off with water.

Firming Face Mask

Ingredients:

2 egg whites separated from yolk

1 tbsp yogurt

Directions:

Whip eggs and yogurt together. Apply mask to face, and leave on for 10 minutes, rinse with warm water.

Honey and Clay Mask

Ingredients:

1 tbsp white clay

1 tbsp honey

1 tsp warm water

1 tsp olive oil

Directions:

Mix clay and honey with a little warm water. Add olive oil and stir.

Apply on face and wash after 20 minutes with cold water.

White Clay Mask

Ingredients:

2 tbsp oats

1 tbsp white clay

3-4 tbsp milk

Directions:

Boil the oatmeal, cool and mix it with 1 tablespoon of clay and a 3-4 tablespoons of milk.

Apply mask to face and rinse off with warm water after 20 minutes.

Lifting Honey and Clay Mask

Ingredients:

1 tbsp honey

2 tbsp lemon juice

1 tbsp white clay

Directions:

Mix ingredients well and apply the mixture to your skin using your fingers.

Cover your face in a thin, even layer and allow to dry for 15 minutes. Wash with cool water.

Anti-aging Red Wine Face Mask

Ingredients:

1 egg white

2 tbsp red wine

1 tbsp honey

Directions:

Mix the egg white, red wine and honey until you have a smooth substance.

Spread the paste with your fingertips on clean face and neck avoiding the eye area. Leave the mask on for 10-15 minutes then wash it off with lukewarm water.

Wheat Bran Mask

Ingredients:

2 tbsp honey

3 tbsp wheat bran.

Directions:

Mix well honey and wheat bran to form a paste and spread on your face. Leave for 30 minutes. Rinse face with warm water.

Peach Mask

Ingredients:

1 ripe peach

1 egg white

Directions:

Whip egg white. Cut the peach and mash it with a fork then stir well with the egg white.

Apply to face and leave for 10 minutes, then wash with cool water.

Peach and Honey Mask

Ingredients:

1 ripe peach

1 tbsp honey

1tbsp oats bran

Directions:

Blend peach and honey in a blender and add oats bran, so you can make it thicker.

Apply to face and rinse after 15 minutes.

Homemade Face Creams and Lotions

This part is not long because sometimes the best solutions are often the simplest, and the least expensive.

The best skin creams and moisturizers for me and my family are just plain **olive oil, almond oil, coconut oil and sesame oil**. (shea and jojoba oils work well too). I'm somewhat breakout-prone so when I started replacing my usual face creams I was worried about slathering oil all over my face. It turned out all these natural oils make me break out far less than any store bought moisturizers (even the expensive ones) and they are so much cheaper.

Coconut Oil and Coconut Butter

I put just a little bit of cocoa oil on my fingertips, while my face is still wet from the shower or washing. It thins out the oil nicely, makes it spread evenly on my face, and it absorbs into my skin faster, with no greasy slick. Coconut has anti-bacterial properties so it also helps heal blemishes and keeps skin clear.

When I researched alternative sunscreens coconut oil came up again, together with sesame oil. And because it turns out that sunscreen actually causes skin cancer - now when I go into the sun or walk the beaches I put on coconut oil. My skin becomes lovely and brown and doesn't burn. (For long periods in intense sun, which I can feel on my skin, I cover up). As a sunscreen it is best to allow the oil to be absorbed in the skin before going out in the direct sun.

Almond Oil

Almond oil is chock full of vitamin E and is great for the skin. It is most suitable for dry or combination skin, but oily skin types like may tolerate it just fine. (Mine does) You just need to try it and see. Use a pea sized amount, and smooth it on your face in upward strokes.

Almond and sesame oils are also fantastic for the skin under and around your eyes. They are ideal for preventing and moisturizing crow's-feet and fine lines. Almond oil has the additional benefit of reducing both dark circles and puffy eyes. Apply one or two drops of oil underneath and around your eyes. Gently pat it using one of your fingers. Do this right before going to bed.

Olive Oil

My favorite beauty "secret" which wasn't a secret to my grandmother is using olive oil on just about every part of my body.

Olive oil is very effective in combating dryness and works wonders on the skin, day or night. If the skin on your face is feeling especially dry, take one or two drops of olive oil in your hands, and very gently tap it all over your face, making sure it doesn't look slick. You can take a tissue and blot your skin just a little. You'll have skin like velvet - soft , but not greasy.

You can use olive oil around your eyes, your lips, hands, nails and cuticles. You can use it to heal insect bites, sun burns and rashes. You can use olive oil to strengthen and nourish your hair and to prevent dandruff. You can also use olive oil for body massage.

Forget expensive skin treatments, fancy moisturizers and other beauty aids. If you want to have glowing, young skin, look no further than your kitchen. Like I already said sometimes the best solutions are also the simplest and easiest!

Best Kept Secrets for Healthy Hair

For the majority of people pampering your hair with homemade shampoos and masks is more time consuming and complicated than using commercial ones. That's why a lot of women don't even try to replace the products they are used to with something they don't know the effects of. Even when they know that shampoos and hair masks are full of harmful chemistry, women still use them because they feel there is no alternative at all.

For many years I too had stopped using homemade hair masks because I either didn't have the time or the will to replace old habits and try something new. Only recently have I started again really thinking what substances I surround myself and my family with, and started eliminating one by one every potentially harmful product in my house. Without being a fanatic, I try to use more natural products in every aspect of our life. That's how I rediscovered homemade hair masks. That, and the fact that I decided to grow long hair again. So after more than a year, I can say that to have and to maintain beautiful, thick and shiny hair is a lot easier than I had initially thought, and it is also very rewarding.

Every woman feels good and happy when she has beautiful hair and the experience of preparing a hair mask at home is actually very exciting and pleasant when you know you are doing it for yourself. You just have to experiment to find out what mask works best for your hair. Try different combinations of ingredients which you think might work for your hair type; adjust the length of time you leave the mask on your hair, and the quantities of each ingredient in the mixture you use. Everybody's hair is different, so your ideal recipe will be unique too. For me, it seems bananas do miracles especially when combined with oatmeal and a little apple cider vinegar. But I am still experimenting and feeding my hair with different masks because it is fun and, if the mask doesn't seem to be the right one, it is no big deal – next time I make something different.

Just remember that healthy hair comes only when we take care of our overall health. There are major steps everyone can follow in order to have healthy, thick and long hair and the most important ones are following a healthy diet with lots of fruit, vegetables, whole grains and proteins, doing enough physical exercise, and, last but not least, getting enough sleep and relaxation.

These recipes are intended for immediate use and therefore do not contain any artificial fragrances, colors or preservatives. However, please be aware that if you have a known food allergy, chances are you will be allergic to a cosmetic product made from the same food. You should always take care when you use a new product - be sure to test a small area of skin for sensitivity before using any mixture on your hair. Dab a little on the inside of your wrist or the underside of your arm and wait for 24 hours to see if it causes a reaction, such as a rash.

Hair Growing Tips

Start with healthy hair

The first and most important step to having long hair is to start with healthy hair. That means something very painful for most of us, but absolutely imperative. You have to remove every cm of hair that is already damaged. If it is damaged it will only get worse as time passes. It is necessary to cut all the split ends once and hope to never do it again. Use very sharp scissors to trim your hair, because using anything else will encourage more splitting. If you are actively growing your hair, trim a cm every three or four months. Bad haircuts can also ruin your hair so finding a good hairdresser is a very good idea.

Always treat wet hair with care

Be especially gentle with your hair when it is wet because wet hair has no elasticity and will snap very easily if it is stretched. One of the most damaging things for the hair is rubbing it vigorously with a towel or brushing it when it is wet (which is exactly what I used to do until a year ago). After washing the hair, squeeze the excess water gently, then wrap your head in a towel, turban-style. Avoid blow dryers and other heated styling tools. Whenever possible, let your hair dry naturally and finish off with a dryer on the lowest setting.

Don't shampoo every day and always wash using warm rather than hot water

If your hair is clean and looks good don't wash it! Washing strips away the natural oils and can irritate the scalp. If you shower more than once a day, use a shower cap. Always use natural shampoos. You can try some of the shampoo recipes in my book and see which one works best for your hair. Then you can start experimenting with replacing every other shampooing with the homemade shampoo. Learn to rinse your hair with water that is as cold as you can take. This makes the hair cuticle lie flat and it is less likely to snag and break so you get the added benefit of very shiny hair that's easier to comb.

Change your shampoo often

Even if you have a favorite shampoo, it is not a good idea to constantly use it. This can cause a residue of particular chemicals to build up in the hair damaging it and making it dull and lifeless. Rotate your brand ever couple of weeks to prevent this - or use a homemade shampoo every other time. Also, it is necessary to purify your hair at least once a month by rinsing it with a mixture of apple cider vinegar and water. This rinse removes the build-up of products in your hair and helps avoid damage to the cuticle. While everyone should purify regularly, this step is absolutely essential if you are using products that contain silicone.

Condition your hair

Conditioners smooth the outer cuticles and seal them to help protect the hair from the damage of combs, brushes and heat, as well as environmental damage. Apply conditioner to the length of the hair after squeezing dry and avoid the scalp if your hair is oily. Leave on for at least two minutes before rinsing off. Comb the conditioner through hair using a wide-tooth comb to make sure it reaches every strand. Try different combinations of natural products like avocado, coconut oil or almond oil, and find out which are best for your hair type. Deep condition your hair at least monthly, even if it's in good shape - this will help keep it that way. If your hair is dry or damaged, deep condition weekly. Hot oil treatments with pure olive or jojoba oil are good alternatives for very dry hair or for extra conditioning. For a really intense conditioning treatment you can try washing and applying conditioner at night, wearing a shower cap to bed, and rinsing your hair in the morning.

Keep combs and brushes clean and choose the right ones for your hair

When you drag a brush or a comb through your hair, all the oils, dirt, bacteria, and dry skin flakes accumulate on it along with the hair you brush out of your head. A natural way to clean combs and brushes is soaking them in a cup of hot water with a teaspoon of baking soda added in it. Do this as often as you wash your hair otherwise you are adding dirt or product residue to clean hair and that reduces its shine. Wash your combs weekly at a minimum.

Protect your hair from the sun

Wear a hat in the sun so that your hair is protected from the damaging effects of both heat and UV rays. If you are doing a lot of swimming then comb UV protection through your hair to avoid damage and drying out your hair. Cold-pressed, unrefined sesame oil acts as a natural sunscreen for hair and protects it from harmful UV rays. The same goes for macadamia oil, which is great for shielding the hair from chemicals, heat and damage through its natural UV protection. If you are going to dip into a chlorine pool or the sea, tie your hair out of the way, and if you swim regularly – use a good swim cap.

Look after your hair while you sleep

Never sleep with hair clipped or tied as you damage and weaken the hair that way. If you toss and turn a lot, braid it loosely to prevent tangles. If at all possible, leave it loose. If possible use a satin pillow case.

What you eat is very important for beautiful hair

What you eat plays a major role in your hair's health and growth. If your body isn't getting enough nutrition, neither is your hair. Make certain you eat a well-balanced diet consisting of all food groups. Eat plenty of fruit, vegetables, whole grains, dairy foods and lean protein to help your hair grow longer and quicker. Be especially careful to get enough protein and iron in your diet. A lack of these nutrients can lead to hair loss. Indulge in foods known for helping your hair grow longer and containing nutrients as the B vitamins, biotin, vitamin E, vitamin C and zinc.

Finding out what foods drive your body best is a key to great success in all areas. Try eating a couple of different dietary programs to find the one that works best for you. It is essential that your body and your hair receive a good and balanced diet. You may feel well on lots of small meals while other people feel better on 2 or 3 bigger meals. Some find their optimal physical success on a high carbohydrate plan while others do better with higher protein levels.

Have realistic expectations about the effect of your dietary changes. Remember that what you eat will not affect the hair that has already grown, but it will affect new growth. Dietary effects on hair may take up to 6 months to become visible even though changing your diet may begin affecting the growth of hair in a much shorter time period.

Relax

Intense physical or emotional stress can cause hair growth to slow or shut down completely. In severe cases, stress can even cause hair loss. The problem is that you use vital nutrients to cope with any stresses on the body and your hair and scalp will lack those. The more you can relax, the better it will be for your hair.

Exercise

Another very important factor for hair growth is exercise. Any type of exercise stimulates the blood circulation, so you can choose what is best for you – walking, running, dancing, yoga, or simply going to the gym or joining an exercise class. Even thirty minutes per day spent exercising are very beneficial.

Nutrition for a Healthy Hair Growth

To maintain beautiful healthy hair and to speed up its growth you should always have in your kitchen the following food groups:

Proteins - Because hair and skin are pure protein, your diet needs to contain live, healthy, protein-based foods. Add protein to your diet by including animal products, such as meat and dairy, or protein shakes made from whey. Making sure you have plenty of protein in your diet will nourish your hair follicles and ensure that they function properly. Other high-protein foods for your diet are eggs, soybeans, fish and legumes. Soy protein has been found to be helpful in stimulating hair growth.

Fatty acids - Certain amounts of fats are good for general health and are necessary for good hair condition. The key is eating the right kinds of fats. Essential fatty acids found in foods such as fish, nuts, spinach, eggs, avocados, pumpkin seeds, flaxseed and walnuts are extremely important for healthy hair. Adding them into your diet will stimulate hair growth and make your hair lustrous. This is so because essential fatty acids nourish your scalp, prevent dandruff and itchiness, and produce natural oils that condition your hair.

B vitamins and biotin - Vitamins B-12, B-6, and biotin will help strengthen your hair's cuticle, the outermost layer. If this layer is strong when it grows out from your scalp, it will stay strong and healthy throughout the hair growth and will not split. Vitamin B-3 helps increase blood circulation to the scalp, thereby encouraging hair growth. For best combination of B vitamins eat bananas, eggs, spinach, salmon, lentils and beans.

Vitamin C is also an important factor for healthy hair growth. Citrus fruits, such as oranges and lemons, are especially high in vitamin C, as are green peppers. Eating these foods will nourish the parts under your scalp that grow the hair. Hair grows about 1.3 cm per month, so you should start to see results in about three to six months, if you start eating these foods now. But be patient.

Iron is a mineral which also helps increase circulation in the scalp, which then fuels hair growth. Foods that are high in iron include liver, apricots, and raisins.

Vitamin A helps create strong, shiny hair because it works with the fat synthesis in the hair follicles and spurs on hair growth. Foods that contain vitamin A include eggs, kale, squash, and carrots.

Vitamin E is another nutrient needed to grow long hair. It stimulates the blood circulation in the scalp and can be taken internally or applied to the scalp. Foods that contain enough vitamin E are avocados, nuts, and seeds.

Raw oats and bean sprouts, green beans and bananas are also beneficial for growing long healthy hair because they contain **silica**, an equally important mineral.

Water makes up one quarter of the hair shaft and you ought to drink at least 4 to 8 cups of water a day to stay hydrated and grow healthy hair.

Centuries-old Tips on How to Use the Moon to Grow Your Hair

During my Mother's and Grandmother's time people always said that it was best to cut your hair between the new moon and first quarter moon. My grandparents always looked through the Lunar calendar for the best days for doing activities. Many gardeners and farmers have been using the moon as a guide to planting and harvesting with documented success for hundreds of years. The pull of the moon is responsible for tidal movements on earth and has an effect on all living things. As we are also composed mainly of water, the moon cycle affects human growth and behavior patterns, hormones and mood swings. Although the hair shaft is technically dead, the moon does have an effect on hair, as hair follicles are made up of tissue mainly composed of hydrogen and oxygen, the two elements that make up water.

The best time to have your hair cut, in order to grow it faster, is right after the new moon when moon light is getting stronger, i.e. when the moon is waxing. You should not cut off a lot: trimming a little bit will work best. The days when the moon is waxing are also beneficial if you are starting a new healthy diet, or other hair care program, intended to get your hair healthier and longer as quickly as possible.

General Rules for Applying Homemade Hair Masks

Prepare your mask. Wash your hair as normal, but don't apply conditioner. Squeeze any excess water out of your hair. Apply your mask evenly through the hair. You can use a wide-toothed comb. Leave the mask for 30-60 minutes, or as indicated in the instructions, and rinse with lukewarm water. Finish with a cool (but not cold) rinse to close the hair follicle.

If you don't want your hair to smell of food, use the mask at night when you don't have to go anywhere until the morning, and if it does smell in the morning, put a few drops of rose water or another natural aroma onto a hairbrush and brush it through your hair.

Aim to apply a mask once or twice a month, more frequent applications can lead to a change of the hair's natural balance, making it greasier or drier.

Basic Ingredients of Homemade Hair Shampoos, Masks and Conditioners

Avocados are one of nature's greatest moisturizers, full of vitamins and nutrients, such as vitamin E and B vitamins, natural oils that give your hair the moisture it's lacking. You can use an avocado, mash it, and comb into hair on its own or mix it with other ingredients to prepare a homemade conditioner or hair mask.

Bananas are rich in vitamins, oils and minerals like silica that are good for improving hair elasticity, and preventing split ends and breakage. They are also good for fighting dandruff. Just make sure the banana is completely mashed and blended and there are no separate pieces of fruit that will be hard to wash away. Combine bananas with avocados, oatmeal, honey or yogurt and find out what combination works best for you.

Honey moisturizes hair and skin and is, therefore, suitable for dry hair. Be aware that it also lightens the color of your hair. Use just a little bit, or, even better, mix it into other ingredients such as avocados, bananas, yogurt or eggs. Apply to damp hair.

Olive oil has been used for centuries to moisturize hair and skin. It is nourishing and strengthening, perfect for dry or damaged hair.

Eggs are full of vitamin D, iron, zinc and a variety of B vitamins, and are very good for strengthening the hair and hair follicles. Eggs are commonly used in hair masks also because of their high levels of protein. Use cool water to remove the egg masks because hot water will scramble the egg in your hair and make it difficult to remove.

Almond oil is a wonderful, natural treatment for dry and damaged hair. It's a good source of vitamin E and essential minerals like magnesium. When applied to the hair, almond oil provides deep nourishment and moisture, adds shine to dull hair, makes hair stronger, controls hair loss and stimulates growth. Apply to slightly wet or damp hair for better absorption on its own or mixed with some other ingredients.

Yogurt is high in lactic acid, and has natural anti-fungal and antibacterial properties. It stimulates hair growth and fights dandruff by acting as a natural cleanser that tightens and clarifies the pores on your scalp. The protein in yogurt helps strengthen and moisturize the hair and the antibacterial ingredients help to soothe the scalp and reduce any itchiness. Use yogurt on its own, or mixed with eggs, avocados, bananas or honey.

Nettles have been used for years to stimulate the growth of hair. They can be picked in the spring or summer and used fresh or dried. Dried nettles can also be bought from a drugstore. Applying a nettle solution to hair and scalp increases blood flow, oxygenates hair follicles, strengthens hair fibers, and promotes healthier, fuller hair. The results of nettle treatments, like with all herbal and natural treatments, do not happen overnight, but continued use eventually produces excellent results.

Rosemary has also been used as a hair tonic for centuries. It has a stimulating action on hair follicles and as hair growth begins in the follicles, adding rosemary to a homemade shampoo or hair mask stimulates the growth and regrowth of hair. Rosemary can be picked and used fresh all summer long or can be bought already dried. I grow my rosemary in a flower pot and have fresh rosemary for cooking and beauty treatments all year long.

Castor oil is used in hair growth masks because of its many curative and medicinal properties. The Ricinoleic acid found in castor oil helps getting rid of bacterial and fungal infections on the scalp that cause hair loss. Regular use of castor oil increases hair growth, reduces damage and breakage, conditions and moisturizes hair and scalp. For best results always use cold-pressed organic castor oil. Apply directly to your scalp and the roots of your hair. Don't rub it through the rest of your hair, as it will be difficult to wash out due to its consistency. It is a good idea to combine a little castor oil with olive, almond or jojoba oil to achieve a lighter and easily applicable solution.

Coconut oil is loaded with Vitamin E and fatty acids which are anti-fungal, anti-oxidizing and anti-bacterial. It can be used as an all-over moisturizer, as a conditioner on its own or combined with other ingredients like avocados or bananas.

Oatmeal is extremely good for hair because it contains lots of B-vitamins, which act as humectants. It is also an excellent film former, sealing in moisture and providing a barrier against environmental hazards. It is a good idea to blend oatmeal very finely after boiling it and before applying it on hair because otherwise it is hard to wash off the little pieces. I sometimes add a tablespoon of ground flaxseed in my hair porridge for even better results.

Burdock root contains a large number of beneficial nutrients including, tannins, inulin, vitamin A and essential fatty acids, and has a long history of use in folk medicine as a blood purifier, diaphoretic and a diuretic. Burdock root infusion and burdock root oil are well known for fighting hair loss and strengthening hair. Making burdock root treatments at home can help maintain a healthy scalp, encourage hair growth and improve hair shine and body. Burdock root should not be used by diabetics or women who are pregnant or breast feeding. You should consult your physician before using burdock oil.

Jojoba oil is an extract of the Jojoba shrub found in California, Arizona and parts of Mexico. Jojoba oil has been used for hundreds of years by Native American to moisturize and grow hair. The molecular makeup of jojoba oil is similar to the natural oils the glands of the scalp produce. Jojoba oil can be applied directly to your hair or mixed in another homemade hair mask to promote hair growth. It is hypoallergenic and will not harm your hair or scalp.

Natural Homemade Shampoos

Baking Soda Wash

Directions:

Stir two tablespoons of baking soda in a cup of water and gently massage your scalp with this.

Rinse it well and finish with an Apple Cider Vinegar Rinse to restore the PH of your scalp. Just stir one tablespoon of vinegar in 2 cups of water and rinse your hair with this.

This is the best hair cleaning method I have found so far. Depending on hair length and type you can experiment with the quantities of baking soda to reach the best one for you.

Egg Yolk Shampoo

Mix two egg yolks with a teaspoon of baking soda and wash hair.

Tea Tree Oil Shampoo

Directions:

Mix one egg yolk with 3 drops of tea tree oil. Wash hair with this mixture and rinse thoroughly with warm water.

Pomegranate Oil Shampoo

Directions:

Mix one egg yolk with one teaspoon pomegranate oil and wash hair.

Lemon and Egg Shampoo

Directions:

Beat one egg and mix it with one tablespoon of lemon juice. Blend it well until smooth, then apply to your hair and scalp massaging for a few minutes. Rinse out with lukewarm water.

Avocado Shampoo

Directions:

Mash one ripe avocado and mix it with one tablespoon of baking soda and one tablespoon water. Mix it well until it reaches a creamy consistence. Massage in hair and rinse out with warm water.

Moisturizing Egg Shampoo

Directions:

Beat well one egg and add one tablespoon of baking soda, two tablespoons lemon juice and one tablespoon olive oil. Stir everything well and massage in hair. Wash out with lukewarm water.

Yogurt Shampoo

Directions:

Mix half a cup yogurt with a teaspoon of baking soda and wash hair with the mixture.

Homemade Hair Treatments that Stimulate Hair Growth

Oatmeal Hair Mask

An oatmeal mask is one of the simplest hair treatments you can make at home with great results.

Directions:

Boil a cup of water and pour it over half a cup of dry oats. Use more, if your hair is long or thick.

Wait for 5 minutes then blend with a blender until there are no little pieces left. Add one tablespoon of almond oil, and a tablespoon of apple cider vinegar. Mix everything together, make sure your hair is combed and dry, and apply the hair mask from root to tip.

Leave it on for an hour or more and wash hair without a shampoo. Oatmeal masks leave hair silky and shiny. Use once a week or every other week.

Burdock Hair Mask

Burdock root oil is used in folk medicine as a herbal remedy for faster hair growth as well as a cure to dandruff and itchy scalp.

Directions:

Wash hair and gently massage burdock oil into wet hair.

Cover with a shower cap and leave for an hour, then rinse with warm water. Do not use this hair treatment if you are pregnant or breastfeeding.

Burdock Root Rinse

When burdock root is infused with hot distilled water it releases the burdock root mucilage well as oils that help the effective recovery of scalp irritation and supply nutrition to the hair follicles. That's probably the reason Burdock Root Rinse is so widely used as a natural aid for hair growth.

Directions:

To make the rinse just boil a teaspoon of dried burdock root in 1 lb water for 5 minutes.

Strain, let cool a little and add a drop of lavender, rosemary or rose oil. Use on washed hair instead of a conditioner. You can mix this infusion with the nettle infusion for better results.

Vitamin A Hair Mask

Directions:

Mix a tablespoon of olive oil, a tablespoon of almond oil and vitamin A ampule. Apply on the whole length of hair, massaging well into roots.

Cover with a shower cap and a warm towel. Leave for an hour and wash well with a mild shampoo.

Mustard Hair Mask

The Mustard Hair Mask is very effective for stimulating healthy hair growth because mustard helps to increase the blood supply to the scalp.

Directions:

Mix one tablespoon of mustard or mustard powder with one egg yolk and a tablespoon of hot water. Apply the mask to roots and hair.

Cover with a shower cap and leave for 15 minutes then wash with shampoo. Use this treatment at least once a week.

Castor Oil Mask

Directions:

Blend a tablespoon of castor oil with a tablespoon of olive oil and heat it moderately. Add it to a beaten egg yolk, stir well and massage onto your scalp with a cotton swab for better application.

Leave it on for an hour. Rinse off with warm water and shampoo.

Rosemary Rinse

Rosemary is a very powerful herb and its regular use on hair makes it soft and shiny while at the same time it stimulates its growth. What rosemary does is bring blood to the scalp and hair roots thus encouraging their growth.

Directions:

Brew a potion using 2 teaspoons of dry or fresh rosemary leaves and 1 1/2 cup of water. Strain and massage the mixture into your hair and scalp starting from the ends. You don't need to rinse it, and you can apply it day. I often combine the rosemary leaves with thyme or lavender leaves for even better results.

Almond Oil Treatment

Another very effective way to grow out and strengthen your hair is treating it with almond oil. Almond oil contains lots of healthy fatty acids and can do miracles for your hair.

Directions:

You can simply massage 1-2 tablespoons of almond oil from hair roots to the ends, leave it on for 15 minutes, then rinse your hair with cool water and shampoo as usual. Or you can mix it with a vitamin A or E ampule and use it that way.

In case of dry or damaged hair, you can do this treatment twice a week. To see results you have to use it for a few weeks, just like with all herbal and natural treatments.

Nettle Hair Rinse

Nettle infusions and masks are probably one of the most used hair growth treatments in Eastern Europe, along with burdock oil masks.

Nettles are incredibly effective if you have thin hair that you're trying to grow out and thicken.

Directions:

For a nettle rinse, boil one cup (1 lb) nettle leaves in two cups of water. Let it simmer on the stove for 10 minutes, then cool and strain it.

Massage the mixture into your scalp every day. For even better results add two tablespoons of apple cider vinegar.

Lemon Juice and Coriander Leaves

A mixture of Lemon Juice and Coriander Leaves has proved to help hair grow faster and is often used to prevent hair loss. Coriander leaves applied to the scalp stimulate faster hair follicle regeneration.

Directions:

Boil half a cup of freshly-squeezed lemon juice and pour it over two tablespoons of chopped fresh coriander leaves.

Let the infusion cool and gently massage into hair roots.

Leave it on for 15 minutes then wash your hair. For best results repeat every day.

Onions for Long Hair

Directions:

Juice a small onion or grate it and strain the liquid. You can either apply the juice all over your hair or add it to a hair mask.

For best results, leave the mask on overnight and shampoo it the next morning. Finish with a Lavender Water Rinse.

Egg and Onion Mask

Directions:

Mix one egg yolk, one teaspoon of honey, one tablespoon of olive oil and two tablespoons of freshly squeezed onion juice. Apply this mask to hair roots, and then spread through the hair.

Cover with a shower cap and a warm towel. Wait for two hours and wash with warm water and shampoo. Apply at least for a few consecutive weeks to see results.

Green Tea and Tea Tree Oil

A common folk remedy for faster hair growth is a mixture of Green Tea and Tea Tree Oil.

Directions:

Boil a cup of water and pour it over a green tea bag. Cover and leave for 5 minutes to cool then add 2 tablespoons of tea tree oil.

Stir well and pour the mixture over the hair and scalp slowly while massaging it. Leave in the hair for 10 to 15 minutes while standing in the shower before rinsing your hair with cool water.

This treatment can be repeated up to three times per day as long as it does not irritate your scalp. You should use only natural tea tree oil because any added ingredients can irritate skin and reduce effectiveness.

Potato and Aloe Vera Hair Mask

Directions:

Peel one potato, grate, and press out the juice. Mix 2 tablespoons of the potato juice with 1 tablespoon aloe vera gel, one vitamin A and one vitamin E capsule and a tablespoon of honey.

Stir well and rub the mixture into hair roots. Cover your hair with a shower cap and wrap it in a towel. Leave for 2 hours then wash your hair with a mild shampoo. Use weekly.

Cinnamon Honey Mask

Directions:

Prepare a hair mask of a tablespoon of honey, an egg yolk, a teaspoon of cinnamon powder and a tablespoon of almond oil.

Warm it very slightly and massage into hair roots and entire hair. Leave the mask for an hour and wash with lukewarm water.

Beer and Egg Hair Mask

Directions:

Mix 1/3 cup beer with an egg yolk. If your hair is long double the beer and use 2 egg yolks. Apply to hair, cover and leave for an hour then wash with lukewarm water.

Egg Yolk and Honey

This mask is used a lot in Eastern Europe and it has very good results.

Directions:

Mix two egg yolks with 2 tablespoons of slightly warmed honey and a tablespoon of almond oil. Stir in a teaspoon of vodka or brandy.

Apply to roots and hair, and cover the head with a shower cap. Leave for 30-40 minutes then wash hair thoroughly, rinsing a couple of times. Use lemon or apple cider water to rinse your hair. Repeat the procedure at least once a month for a few months.

Treatments to Get Rid of Dandruff

Thyme Dandruff Treatment

Directions:

Mix a teaspoon of thyme oil with two tablespoons of almond oil. Warm slightly, massage into scalp and leave for 20 minutes. Wash using a mild shampoo and rinse with cool water.

Thyme Hair Rinse

Directions:

Boil 3 tablespoons of dried thyme into 1 cup of water for 10 minutes. Strain the infusion and leave it to cool. Rinse hair with this daily. Don't wash out.

Strawberry Dandruff Mask

Strawberries are rich in salicilic acid which is very good for fighting dandruff.

Directions:

Mash a few strawberries until a smooth paste is formed then add two or three drops of tea tree oil, rosemary oil or peppermint oil. Apply the mask to washed hair and leave for an hour.

Camphor Oil Mask for Dandruff

Camphor is a herbal substance derived from the camphor tree. When camphor oil is added to a hair mask, it can treat viral conditions or bacterial and fungal infections of the scalp.

Directions:

To cure dandruff, mix a few drops of camphor oil in some coconut oil or jojoba oil, or even a tablespoon of olive oil and massage into your hair and scalp.

Do it at least several times to see results.

Camphor Rinse

Directions:

Another good dandruff treatment is a final rinse prepared from a cup of rosemary or thyme tea with two-three drops of camphor oil in it.

Coconut Lemon Mask

Directions:

Mix two tablespoons of lemon or lime juice with four tablespoons of slightly warmed coconut oil and massage this into your scalp.

Leave it in for a few hours or overnight and wash it out with cool water the next morning. Apply at least once a week.

Ginger Dandruff Treatment

Directions:

Mix one tablespoon of ginger juice, one teaspoon of lime juice and two drops of tea tree oil.

Massage into hair roots and let dry before shampooing. Apply at least twice a week.

The Best Homemade Hair Masks

Masks for Dry Hair

Dry hair usually looks dull, has split ends, and breaks easily. It can be the result of chemical damage or just insufficient oil production. Dry hair always looks the same after you wash it as it did before.

Warm Oil Treatment

Directions:

One of the best treatments for dry hair is Warm Oil Treatment. You need about 3 tablespoons of some basic oil like extra virgin olive oil, jojoba or coconut oil.

For hair that is medium length, 3 tablespoons of oil are enough, but you can use more or less depending on your hair texture and length.

Wrap a towel around neck and shoulders and divide hair into small sections. Heat the oil gently but don't make it too warm. Stir in about 5 drops of lavender, rose, sandalwood, chamomile or tea tree oil to add a pleasant scent and moisture to hair.

Apply on dry hair with a fine-toothed comb making sure to get to the tips. Wrap hair in plastic wrap or wear a shower cap and leave it for 30 minutes. Then shampoo once or twice.

Nourishing Cocoa Mask

Directions:

Slightly warm two tablespoons of honey and stir in two tablespoons of cocoa powder. Add an egg yolk and a tablespoon of almond or olive oil.

Cover neck and shoulders with a towel and apply the mask to dry hair. Cover with a shower cap and a towel and leave at for at least two hours then wash well with shampoo.

Coconut Mask

Coconut oil mixed with a mashed avocado adds shine to your hair and helps scalp get rid of dandruff.

Directions:

Heat the coconut oil very slightly, then mix it with the avocado.

Apply to the hair massaging from the roots to the tips. Leave the mask for 10 to 15 minutes, then use cool water to rinse it.

Simple Dry Hair Banana Mask

Directions:

The easiest banana mask is to blend a ripe banana with a tablespoon of almond oil, coconut or olive oil or just to mix it with a vitamin E or A capsule and when it is smooth and creamy to apply to dry hair for half an hour.

Wash with warm water and shampoo.

Sweet Banana Mask

Directions:

Blend very well one banana with a blender or a hand mixer. Add a tablespoon of honey, one egg yolk and a tablespoon of olive oil. Mix it until it becomes smooth and creamy. Add a vitamin E or A capsule for extra nourishment.

Spread the mixture through your hair and leave it on for 15 to 30 minutes.

Banana Avocado Hair Mask

Directions:

Blend a banana and a ripe avocado until the mixture turns to a creamy consistency. Add a drop of rose essential oil or rosemary oil and apply the mixture to your hair beginning at the scalp and working down to the ends.

Leave on for 30 minutes. Wash thoroughly with a mild shampoo.

Avocado Dry Hair Mask

Directions:

Mash a ripe avocado with a teaspoon of honey, and a teaspoon of olive oil. Apply to hair, leave it on for 30 minutes, then rinse and wash.

Dry Hair Egg Mask

Directions:

Mix 2 egg yolks with a tablespoon of castor oil and a tablespoon of almond oil. Dilute the mixture by adding one tablespoon of warm water or rosemary infusion and then slowly and thoroughly massage this mask into your scalp.

Cover your head with a shower cap and leave it on for at least 30 minutes for the oil to penetrate into your hair. Wash off with a shampoo.

Masks for Oily Hair

Oily hair tends to become greasy if not washed daily and loses its shine throughout the day. The great advantage of making your own hair masks especially in this case, is that the ingredients in homemade masks care for and feed the scalp and hair without drying them out.

Use oily hair masks only once a month to avoid taking away too much oil from the scalp, because in that case it starts to overproduce oil and hair condition becomes worse. Don't over-wash the hair and do not over-brush limp hair since this can stimulate more sebum production.

Basic Mask for Oily Hair

Directions:

A very Basic Mask for Oily Hair is an egg white beaten and mixed with a teaspoon of salt and the juice of half a lemon. Leave the mask on your hair for a half hour and then rinse and wash with a gentle shampoo.

Baking Soda Mask

Baking soda is an effective ingredient for removing build-up of cosmetic products, grease and dirt from the hair.

Directions:

Add a teaspoon to ½ cup mayonnaise or yogurt, and then apply to hair for 30 minutes. Wash only with water.

Yogurt Mask for Oily Hair

Directions:

Whip an egg white and stir it in a cup of yogurt. Add a teaspoon of baking soda and apply to dry hair. Leave for about 40 minutes. Wash with cool water only, because of the egg white.

Honey and Apple Cider Mask for Oily Hair

Apple cider helps remove any build-up of oil from the hair.

Directions:

Mix one tablespoon of slightly warmed honey with three tablespoons of apple cider vinegar. Whisk in 2-3 drops rosemary or lavender essential oil and mix well.

Wet your hair, and then pat it with a towel to remove excess water. Massage the mask into your hair starting from the roots and working down to the tips. Allow the mask to remain in your hair for 15 to 20 minutes then shampoo with warm water.

Strawberry Hair Mask for Oily Hair

Strawberries are good for regulating oil production in the scalp and removing any oil from your hair. They are also full of vitamin C, and have salicylic acid which is good for fighting dandruff.

Directions:

Mash a few strawberries, add 2 tablespoons of yogurt and massage into hair.

Leave on for just 10 minutes to prevent hair from over-drying.

Avocado Mask for Oily Hair

Directions:

Mash one ripe avocado with a tablespoon of fresh lemon or lime juice and one tablespoon aloe vera juice or gel. Apply to hair, cover and leave for 30 minutes, then wash with warm water.

Simple Clay Mask

When using any type of clay put it in a wooden, ceramic or glass bowl and use a wooden spoon or your fingers to manipulate it.

With clay masks results begin to show after the first few weeks, just like with all the other natural and herbal treatments.

Directions:

Mix about 2-4 tablespoons of white clay with a little bit of water. Add half a teaspoon almond oil. Massage into your scalp and hair until all hair is covered.

Leave it on for 30 minutes and then rinse with lots of water and a mild shampoo. It is good to do a final rinse using lemon water or Apple Cider Vinegar Rinse.

Egg Yolk and Clay Mask for Oily Hair

This clay mask gives amazing results for oily hair and also treats hair loss.

Directions:

Mix 2 tablespoons of clay with one egg yolk and a little bit of water. Massage your scalp and hair with the mask and leave on for 30 minutes.

Wash with lots of water and a gentle shampoo. Rinse with lemon water or apple cider vinegar rinse.

Nettle Rinse

Nettles have been used in Bulgaria for more than thousand years to treat a large number of health conditions but are especially effective for stopping hair loss and obtaining healthy and strong hair.

This nettle infusion improves blood circulation in the skin of the scalp and in this way helps hair grow faster and stronger. It also has a long-lasting degreasing effect on hair.

Directions:

Soak a cup of finely cut nettle leaves or roots in two cups of water for a couple of hours or leave them overnight.

Boil everything for 5 minutes, cool, strain, and massage into hair. It is best to do it every day for at least a month. Nettle leaves and roots can be found in most health stores.

Walnut Leaves Rinse

Walnut leaves are a great remedy for oily hair and have been used for hundreds of years in many cultures as they have astringent, antifungal, antibacterial, and calming properties.

Directions:

Take about 10-15 walnut leaves and boil them for 10 minutes in 1 liter of water. Leave to cool down, strain, and you use this water to rinse your hair after you wash it. Repeat this treatment at least twice a week for long lasting effect.

Caution should be taken by people who don't want to change their hair color. Walnut leaves give a dark tint to hair and many women use them to make their hair darker.

Lavender Water Rinse

Lavender leaves have many therapeutic properties along with their powerful aroma. They have long been known for their anti-depressive, antiseptic, astringent, decongestant and anti-rheumatic properties and can a treat a lot of health conditions, including oily hair.

Directions:

Soak 10-15 lavender leaves in 1 liter of water. Leave them for a whole night then boil them. Strain the concoction and use it to rinse your hair after each wash.

Apple Cider Vinegar Rinse

Apple cider vinegar contains nutrients which make hair stronger, shinier and healthier. It also removes any residues from cosmetic products. Apple cider vinegar regulates the pH of the scalp so it is also a good dandruff remedy.

Directions:

To prepare the rinse, dilute 1 part vinegar to 2/3 parts water.

Coffee or Black Tea Hair Rinse

Directions:

Make a good strong espresso, or a strong black tea, leave it to cool and use it as a final hair rinse. The tannins in tea and coffee will dry and regulate the oil production of your scalp. Do not use this on very light hair, and do not use instant coffee.

Masks for Combination Hair

Combination hair tends to be oily at the roots, but dry and damaged towards the ends. This type of problem is often due to over-styling. Hair masks for oily hair are also beneficial for combination hair but have to be applied only to the roots of the hair. When you finish washing the hair always comb the hair ends with a few drops of almond oil, coconut oil, wheat germ oil, grape-seeds oil, shea or jojoba oils.

Masks for Normal Hair

Normal hair doesn't have many problems, usually looks shiny, without many split ends, and is easy to manage. If you want your normal hair to be healthy and long, you will benefit from these homemade hair masks:

Milk and Honey Mask

Directions:

Mix two tablespoons of honey with half a cup of slightly warmed full-fat milk and apply evenly on hair. Cover with a shower cap and leave for half an hour then wash off with a mild shampoo.

A Nourishing Normal Hair Mask

Directions:

Mix two tablespoons of honey, one tablespoon of almond oil and one tablespoon of apple cider vinegar. Apply to the roots before washing your hair and comb through. Leave the mask on for an hour, then rinse it out.

Beer Treatment for Normal Hair

Beer is made from malt and hops, which contain proteins and sugars and are believed to repair hair damaged by chemical processing, sun, chlorine and pollution. Beer is also believed to make hair shiny by tightening the hair cuticles.

Directions:

Blend one banana until completely smooth and mix in one egg. Add ½ cup of flat beer and blend some more. Apply to scalp, roots and all the hair to the ends. Leave the mask for a few hours, and then shampoo out.

Beer Rinse

Directions:

Mix half a cup of flat beer and half a cup of apple cider vinegar. Apply to hair after shampooing, leave for a few minutes then rinse with cool water. It will act like a wonderful conditioner and will give shine to your hair.

Regenerating Mask

Directions:

Beat an egg yolk with a few drops of vitamin A, vitamin E and a teaspoon of castor oil. Add a teaspoon of brandy and stir.

Apply the mixture to your scalp and gently massage in. Leave the mask for two hours and wash your hair with a mild shampoo. Use twice a month for best regenerating effects.

Coconut Oil Mask

Directions:

When applied on wet hair, coconut oil can do wonders for its shine, health and volume. You can also use a very small amount of coconut oil on the ends of your hair after showering as a detangler and as a daily moisturizer.

Clay Mask for Normal Hair

Directions:

Mix two tablespoons of white clay with two tablespoons of olive oil, an egg yolk and a tablespoon of brandy or vodka. Stir well and apply to dry hair.

Cover with a shower cap and leave for an hour then wash with shampoo.

About the Author

Vesela lives in Bulgaria with her family of six (including the Jack Russell Terrier). Her passion is going green in everyday life and she loves to prepare homemade cosmetic and beauty products for all her family and friends.

Vesela has been publishing her cookbooks for over a year now. If you want to see other healthy family recipes that she has published, together with some natural beauty books, you can check out her [Author Page](#) on Amazon.

Manufactured by Amazon.ca
Bolton, ON